The Keto Seafood Cookbook

A Comprehensive Cooking Guide for Delicious Keto Seafood Recipes

By Carla Wilson

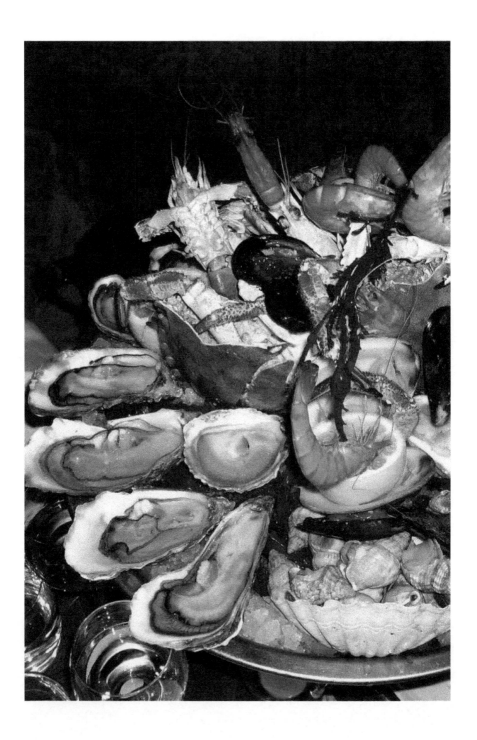

content within this book has been derived from various sources. Please consult a licensed professional before attempting any techniques outlined in this book.

By reading this document, the reader agrees that under no circumstances is the author responsible for any losses, direct or indirect, which are incurred as a result of the use of information contained within this document, including, but not limited to, — errors, omissions, or inaccuracies.

Table of Contents

Mahi-Mahi Taco Wraps

Preparation Time: 5 minutes

Cooking Time: 2 hours

Servings: 6

Ingredients:

- 1-pound Mahi-Mahi, wild-caught
- ½ cup cherry tomatoes
- 1 small green bell pepper, cored and sliced
- 1/4 of a medium red onion, thinly sliced
- ½ teaspoon garlic powder
- 1 teaspoon sea salt
- ½ teaspoon ground black pepper
- 1 teaspoon chipotle pepper
- ½ teaspoon dried oregano
- 1 teaspoon cumin
- 2 tablespoons avocado oil
- 1/4 cup chicken stock
- 1 medium avocado, diced
- 1 cup sour cream
- 6 large lettuce leaves

Directions:

1. Grease a 6-quarts slow cooker with oil, place fish in it and then pour in chicken stock. Stir together garlic powder, salt, black pepper, chipotle pepper, oregano and cumin and then season fish with half of this mixture.
2. Layer fish with tomatoes, pepper and onion, season with remaining spice mixture and shut with lid.
3. Plug in the slow cooker and cook fish for 2 hours at high heat setting or until cooked through. When done, evenly spoon fish among lettuce, top with avocado and sour cream and serve.

Nutrition:

- 193.6g Calories
- 12g Total Fat
- 17g Protein
- 3g Fiber

Shrimp Scampi

Preparation Time: 5 minutes

Cooking Time: 2 hours and 30 minutes

Servings: 4

Ingredients:

- 1 pound wild-caught shrimps, peeled & deveined
- 1 tablespoon minced garlic
- 1 teaspoon salt
- ½ teaspoon ground black pepper
- 1/2 teaspoon red pepper flakes
- 2 tablespoons chopped parsley
- 2 tablespoons avocado oil
- 2 tablespoons unsalted butter
- 1/2 cup white wine
- 1 tablespoon lemon juice
- 1/4 cup chicken broth
- ½ cup grated parmesan cheese

Directions:

1. Place all the ingredients except for shrimps and cheese in a 6-quart slow cooker and whisk until combined.
2. Add shrimps and stir until evenly coated and shut with lid.

3. Plug in the slow cooker and cook for 1 hour and 30 minutes to 2 hours and 30 minutes at low heat setting or until cooked through. Then top with parmesan cheese and serve.

Nutrition:

- 234 Calories
- 14.7g Total Fat
- 23.3g Protein

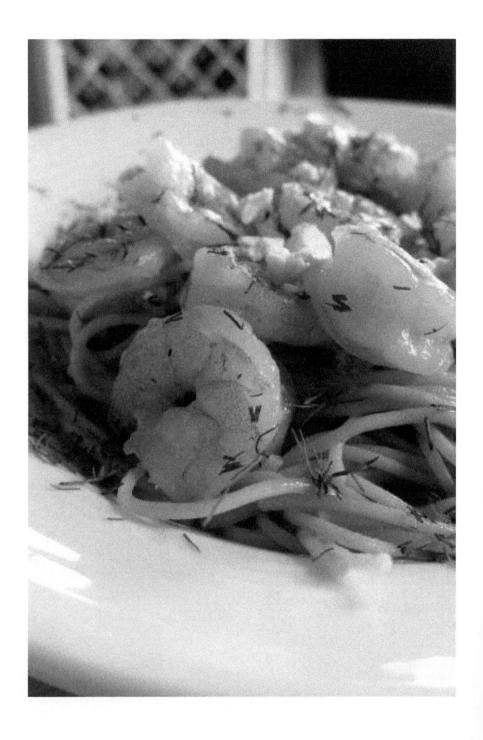

Shrimp Tacos

Preparation Time: 5 minutes

Cooking Time: 3 hours

Servings: 6

Ingredients:

- 1 pound medium wild-caught shrimp, peeled and tails off
- 12-ounce fire-roasted tomatoes, diced
- 1 small green bell pepper, chopped
- ½ cup chopped white onion
- 1 teaspoon minced garlic
- ½ teaspoon sea salt
- ½ teaspoon ground black pepper
- ½ teaspoon red chili powder
- ½ teaspoon cumin
- ¼ teaspoon cayenne pepper
- 2 tablespoons avocado oil
- 1/2 cup salsa
- 4 tablespoons chopped cilantro
- 1 ½ cup sour cream
- 2 media avocados, diced

Directions:

1. Rinse shrimps, layer into a 6-quarts slow cooker and drizzle with oil. Add tomatoes, stir until mixed, then add peppers and remaining ingredients except for sour cream and avocado and stir until combined.
2. Plug in the slow cooker, shut with lid and cook for 2 to 3 hours at low heat setting or 1 hour and 30 minutes to 2 hours at high heat setting or until shrimps turn pink. When done, serve shrimps with avocado and sour cream.

Nutrition:

- 369 Calories
- 27.5g Total Fat
- 21.2g Protein

Fish Curry

Preparation Time: 5 minutes

Cooking Time: 4 hours and 30 minutes

Servings: 6

Ingredients:

- 12 pounds wild-caught white fish fillet, cubed
- 18-ounce spinach leaves
- 4 tablespoons red curry paste, organic
- 14-ounce coconut cream, unsweetened and full-fat
- 14-ounce water

Directions:

1. Plug in a 6-quart slow cooker and let preheat at high heat setting. In the meantime, whisk together coconut cream and water until smooth.

2. Place fish into the slow cooker, spread with curry paste and then pour in coconut cream mixture. Shut with lid and cook for 2 hours at high heat setting or 4 hours at low heat setting until tender.

3. Then add spinach and continue cooking for 20 to 30 minutes or until spinach leaves wilt. Serve straightaway.

Nutrition:

- 323 Calories
- 51.5g Total Fat
- 41.3g Protein

Salmon with Creamy Lemon Sauce

Preparation Time: 5 minutes

Cooking Time: 2 hours and 15 minutes

Servings: 6

Ingredients:

For the Salmon:

- 2 pounds wild-caught salmon fillet, skin-on
- 1 teaspoon garlic powder
- 1 ½ teaspoon salt
- 1 teaspoon ground black pepper
- 1/2 teaspoon red chili powder
- 1 teaspoon Italian Seasoning
- 1 lemon, sliced
- 1 lemon, juiced
- 2 tablespoons avocado oil
- 1 cup chicken broth

For the Creamy Lemon Sauce:

- Chopped parsley, for garnish
- 1/8 teaspoon lemon zest
- 1/4 cup heavy cream
- 1/4 cup grated parmesan cheese

Directions:

1. Line a 6-quart slow cooker with parchment sheet, spread its bottom with lemon slices, then top with salmon and drizzle with oil. Stir together garlic powder, salt, black pepper, red chili powder, Italian seasoning, and oil until combined and rub this mixture all over salmon.

2. Pour lemon juice and broth around the fish and shut with lid. Plug in the slow cooker and cook for 2 hours at low heat setting. In the meantime, set the oven at 400 degrees F and let preheat.

3. When fish is done, lift out an inner pot of slow cooker, place into the oven and cook for 5 to 8 minutes or until top is nicely browned. Lift out fish using parchment sheet and keep it warm.

4. Transfer juices from slow cooker to a medium skillet pan, place it over medium-high heat, then bring to boil and cook for 1 minute. Turn heat to a low level, whisk cream into the sauce along with lemon zest and parmesan cheese and cook for 2 to 3 minutes or until thickened. Cut salmon in pieces, then top each piece with lemon sauce and serve.

Nutrition:

- 340 Calories
- 20g Total Fat
- 32g Protein

Salmon with Lemon-Caper Sauce

Preparation Time: 5 minutes

Cooking Time: 1 hour and 30 minutes

Servings: 4

Ingredients:

- 1 pound wild-caught salmon fillet
- 2 teaspoon capers, rinsed and mashed
- 1 teaspoon minced garlic
- 1 teaspoon salt
- ½ teaspoon ground black pepper
- 1/2 teaspoon dried oregano
- 1 teaspoon lemon zest
- 2 tablespoons lemon juice
- 4 tablespoons unsalted butter

Directions:

1. Cut salmon into 4 pieces, then season with salt and black pepper and sprinkle lemon zest on top.
2. Line a 6-quart slow cooker with parchment paper, place seasoned salmon pieces on it and shut with lid.
3. Plug in the slow cooker and cook for 1 hour and 30 minutes or until salmon is cooked through. When 10 minutes of cooking time is left, prepare lemon-caper

sauce and for this, place a small saucepan over low heat, add butter and let it melt.

4. Then add capers, garlic, lemon juice, stir until mixed and simmer for 1 minute. Remove saucepan from heat and stir in oregano. When salmon is cooked, spoon lemon-caper sauce on it and serve.

Nutrition:

- 368.5 Calories
- 26.6g Total Fat
- 19.5g Protein

Spicy Barbecue Shrimp

Preparation Time: 5 minutes

Cooking Time: 1 hour and 30 minutes

Servings: 6

Ingredients:

- 1 1/2 pounds large wild-caught shrimp, unpeeled
- 1 green onion, chopped
- 1 teaspoon minced garlic
- 1 ½ teaspoon salt
- ¾ teaspoon ground black pepper
- 1 teaspoon Cajun seasoning
- 1 tablespoon hot pepper sauce
- ¼ cup Worcestershire Sauce
- 1 lemon, juiced
- 2 tablespoons avocado oil
- 1/2 cup unsalted butter, chopped

Directions:

1. Place all the ingredients except for shrimps in a 6-quart slow cooker and whisk until mixed.
2. Plug in the slow cooker, then shut with lid and cook for 30 minutes at high heat setting. Then take out ½ cup of this sauce and reserve. Add shrimps to slow cooker.

Nutrition:

- 321 Calories
- 21.4g Total Fat
- 27.3g Protein

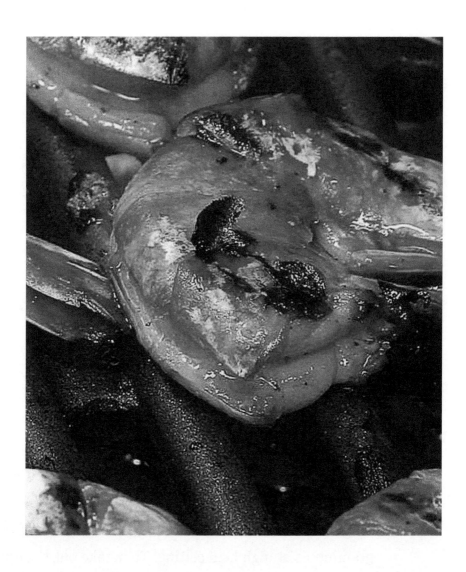

Lemon Dill Halibut

Preparation Time: 5 minutes

Cooking Time: 2 hours

Servings: 2

Ingredients:

- 12-ounce wild-caught halibut fillet
- 1 teaspoon salt
- ½ teaspoon ground black pepper
- 1 1/2 teaspoon dried dill
- 1 tablespoon fresh lemon juice
- 3 tablespoons avocado oil

Directions:

1. Cut an 18-inch piece of aluminum foil, place halibut fillet in the middle and then season with salt and black pepper. Whisk together remaining ingredients, drizzle this mixture over halibut, then crimp the edges of foil and place it into a 6-quart slow cooker.

2. Plug in the slow cooker, shut with lid and cook for 1 hour and 30 minutes or 2 hours at high heat setting or until cooked through. When done, carefully open the crimped edges and check the fish, it should be tender and flaky. Serve straightaway.

Nutrition:

- 321.5 Calories
- 21.4g Total Fat
- 32.1g Protein

Coconut Cilantro Curry Shrimp

Preparation Time: 5 minutes

Cooking Time: 2 hours and 30 minutes

Servings: 4

Ingredients:

- 1 pound wild-caught shrimp, peeled and deveined
- 2 ½ teaspoon lemon garlic seasoning
- 2 tablespoons red curry paste
- 4 tablespoons chopped cilantro
- 30 ounces coconut milk, unsweetened
- 16 ounces water

Directions:

1. Whisk together all the ingredients except for shrimps and 2 tablespoons cilantro and add to a 4-quart slow cooker. Plug in the slow cooker, shut with lid and cook for 2 hours at high heat setting or 4 hours at low heat setting.

2. Then add shrimps, toss until evenly coated and cook for 20 to 30 minutes at high heat settings or until shrimps are pink. Garnish shrimps with remaining cilantro and serve.

Nutrition:

- 160.7 Calories
- 8.2g Total Fat
- 19.3g Protein

Shrimp in Marinara Sauce

Preparation Time: 5 minutes

Cooking Time: 5 hours and 10 minutes

Servings: 5

Ingredients:

- 1 pound cooked wild-caught shrimps, peeled and deveined
- 14.5-ounce crushed tomatoes
- ½ teaspoon minced garlic
- 1 teaspoon salt
- 1/2 teaspoon seasoned salt
- ¼ teaspoon ground black pepper
- ½ teaspoon crushed red pepper flakes
- 1/2 teaspoon dried basil
- 1/2 teaspoon dried oregano
- ½ tablespoons avocado oil
- 6-ounce chicken broth
- 2 tablespoon minced parsley
- 1/2 cup grated Parmesan cheese

Directions:

1. Place all the ingredients except for shrimps, parsley, and cheese in a 4-quart slow cooker and stir well. Then

plug in the slow cooker, shut with lid and cook for 4 to 5 hours at low heat setting.

2. Then add shrimps and parsley, stir until mixed and cook for 10 minutes at high heat setting. Garnish shrimps with cheese and serve.

Nutrition:

- 358.8 Calories
- 25.1g Total Fat
- 26g Protein

Garlic Shrimp

Preparation Time: 5 minutes

Cooking Time: 1 hour

Servings: 5

Ingredients:

For the Garlic Shrimp:

- 1 1/2 pounds large wild-caught shrimp, peeled and deveined
- 1/4 teaspoon ground black pepper
- 1/8 teaspoon ground cayenne pepper
- 2 ½ teaspoons minced garlic
- 1/4 cup avocado oil
- 4 tablespoons unsalted butter

For the Seasoning:

- 1 teaspoon onion powder
- 1 tablespoon garlic powder
- 1 tablespoon salt
- 2 teaspoons ground black pepper
- 1 tablespoon paprika
- 1 teaspoon cayenne pepper
- 1 teaspoon dried oregano
- 1 teaspoon dried thyme

Directions:

1. Stir together all the ingredients for seasoning, garlic, oil, and butter and add to a 4-quart slow cooker. Plug in the slow cooker, shut with lid and cook for 25 to 30 minutes at high heat setting or until cooked.
2. Then add shrimps, toss until evenly coated and continue cooking for 20 to 30 minutes at high heat setting or until shrimps are pink. When done, transfer shrimps to a serving plate, top with sauce and serve.

Nutrition:

- 233.6 Calories
- 11.7g Total Fat
- 30.9g Protein

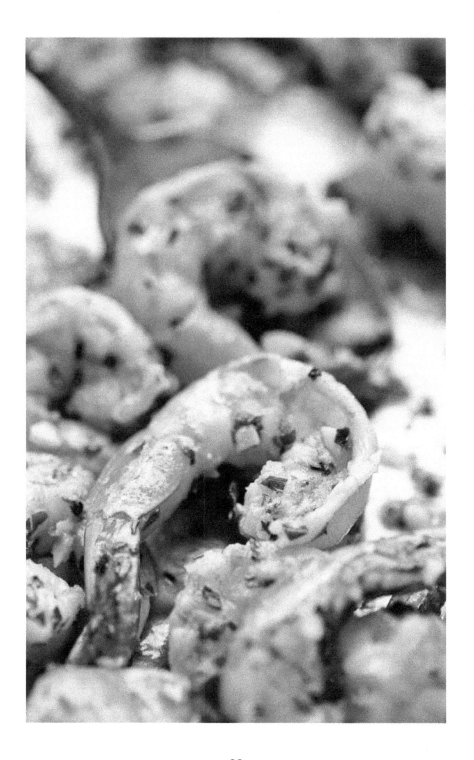

Poached Salmon

Preparation Time: 5 minutes

Cooking Time: 3 hours and 35 minutes

Servings: 4

Ingredients:

- 4 steaks of wild-caught salmon
- 1 medium white onion, peeled and sliced
- 2 teaspoons minced garlic
- 1/2 teaspoon salt
- 1/8 teaspoon ground white pepper
- 1/2 teaspoon dried dill weed
- 2 tablespoons avocado oil
- 2 tablespoons unsalted butter
- 2 tablespoons lemon juice
- 1 cup water

Directions:

1. Place butter in a 4-quart slow cooker, then add salmon and drizzle with oil. Place remaining ingredients in a medium saucepan, stir until mixed and bring the mixture to boil over high heat.

2. Then pour this mixture all over salmon and shut with lid. Plug in the slow cooker and cook salmon for 3

hours and 30 minutes at low heat setting or until salmon is tender. Serve straightaway.

Nutrition:

- 310 Calories
- 20g Total Fat
- 30.2g Protein

Lemon Pepper Tilapia

Preparation Time: 5 minutes

Cooking Time: 3 hours

Servings: 6

Ingredients:

- 6 wild-caught Tilapia fillets
- 4 teaspoons lemon-pepper seasoning, divided
- 6 tablespoons unsalted butter, divided
- 1/2 cup lemon juice, fresh

Directions:

1. Cut a large piece of aluminum foil for each fillet and then arrange them on a clean working space. Place each fillet in the middle of the foil, then season with lemon-pepper seasoning, drizzle with lemon juice and top with 1 tablespoon butter.

2. Gently crimp the edges of foil to form a packet and place it into a 6-quart slow cooker. Plug in the slow cooker, shut with lid and cook for 3 hours at high heat setting or until cooked through.

3. When done, carefully remove packets from the slow cooker and open the crimped edges and check the fish, it should be tender and flaky. Serve straightaway.

Nutrition:

- 201.1 Calories
- 12.9g Total Fat
- 19.6g Protein

Clam Chowder

Preparation Time: 5 minutes

Cooking Time: 6 hours

Servings: 6

Ingredients:

- 20-ounce wild-caught baby clams, with juice
- ½ cup chopped scallion
- ½ cup chopped celery
- 1 teaspoon salt
- 1 teaspoon ground black pepper
- 1 teaspoon dried thyme
- 1 tablespoon avocado oil
- 2 cups coconut cream, full-fat
- 2 cups chicken broth

Directions:

1. Grease a 6-quart slow cooker with oil, then add ingredients and stir until mixed. Plug in the slow cooker, shut with lid and cook for 4 to 6 hours at low heat setting or until cooked through. Serve straightaway.

Nutrition:

- 357 Calories
- 28.9g Total Fat
- 15.2g Protein

Soy-Ginger Steamed Pompano

Preparation Time: 5 minutes

Cooking Time: 1 hour

Servings: 4

Ingredients:

- 1 wild-caught whole pompano, gutted and scaled
- 1 bunch scallion, diced
- 1 bunch cilantro, chopped
- 3 teaspoons minced garlic
- 1 tablespoon grated ginger
- 1 tablespoon swerve sweetener
- ¼ cup soy sauce
- ¼ cup white wine
- ¼ cup sesame oil

Directions:

1. Place scallions in a 6-quart slow cooker and top with fish. Whisk together remaining ingredients, except for cilantro, and pour the mixture all over the fish.
2. Plug in the slow cooker, shut with lid and cook for 1 hour at high heat setting or until cooked through. Garnish with cilantro and serve

Nutrition:

- 202.5 Calories
- 24.2g Total Fat
- 22.7g Protein

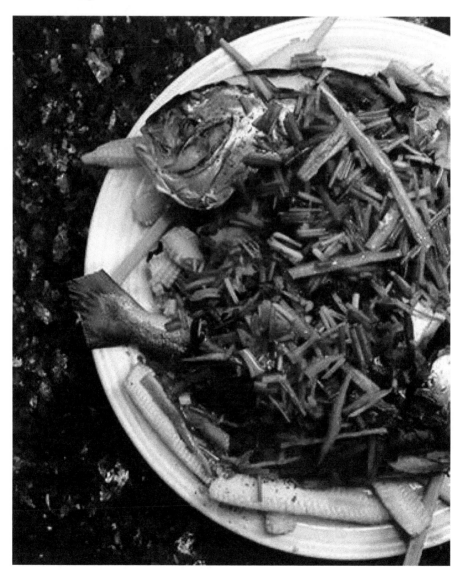

Keto Salmon Tandoori with Cucumber Sauce

Preparation Time: 10 minutes

Cooking Time: 20 minutes

Servings: 4

Ingredients:

- 25 ounces salmon
- Two tablespoons coconut oil
- One tablespoon tandoori seasoning

For the cucumber sauce:

- 1/2 shredded cucumber
- Juice of 1/2 lime
- Two minced garlic cloves
- 1 1/4 cups sour cream

For the crispy salad:

- 3 1/2 ounces lettuce
- Three scallions
- Two avocados
- One yellow bell pepper
- Juice of 1 lime

Directions:

1. Preheat the oven to 350 degrees Fahrenheit
2. Mix the tandoori seasoning with oil and coat the salmon pieces with this mixture.
3. Bake for 20 minutes
4. Place the shredded cucumber in it. Add the mayonnaise, minced garlic, and salt to the shredded cucumber.
5. Mix the lettuce, scallions, avocados, and bell pepper. Drizzle the contents with the lime juice.
6. Transfer the veggie salad to a plate and place the baked salmon over it. Top with cucumber sauce.

Nutrition:

- 847 Calories
- 73g Fat
- 35g Protein

Creamy Mackerel

Preparation Time: 10 minutes

Cooking Time: 20 minutes

Servings: 4

Ingredients:

- Two shallots
- Two spring onions
- Two tablespoons olive oil
- Four mackerel fillets
- 1 cup heavy cream
- One teaspoon cumin
- ½ teaspoon oregano
- Two tablespoons chives

Directions:

1. Preheat pan with the oil over medium heat, sauté spring onions and the shallots for 5 minutes.
2. Cook fish for 4 minutes.
3. Simmer the rest of the ingredients for 10 minutes more, and serve.

Nutrition:

- 403 Calories
- 33.9g Fat
- 22g Protein

Lime Mackerel

Preparation Time: 10 minutes

Cooking Time: 30 Minutes

Servings: 4

Ingredients:

- Four mackerel fillets
- Two tablespoons lime juice
- Two tablespoons olive oil
- ½ teaspoon sweet paprika

Directions:

1. Arrange the mackerel on a baking sheet lined with parchment paper, add the oil and the other ingredients, rub gently, and bake at 360 degrees F for 30 minutes.

Nutrition:

- 297 Calories
- 22.7g Fat
- 0.2g Fiber

Turmeric Tilapia

Preparation Time: 10 minutes

Cooking Time: 12 minutes

Servings: 4

Ingredients:

- Four tilapia fillets
- Two tablespoons olive oil
- One teaspoon turmeric powder
- Two spring onions
- ¼ teaspoon basil
- ¼ teaspoon garlic powder
- One tablespoon parsley

Directions:

1. Cook oil over medium heat, cook the spring onions for 2 minutes.
2. Cook fish, turmeric, and the other ingredients for 5 minutes on each side, and serve.

Nutrition:

- 205 Calories
- 8.6g Fat
- 0.4g Fiber

Walnut Salmon Mix

Preparation Time: 10 minutes

Cooking Time: 14 minutes

Servings: 4

Ingredients:

- Four salmon fillets
- Two tablespoons avocado oil
- One tablespoon lime juice
- Two shallots, chopped
- Two tablespoons walnuts
- Two tablespoons parsley

Directions:

1. Heat up oil over medium-high heat, sauté the shallots.
2. Add the fish and the other ingredients, cook for 6 minutes on each side, and serve.

Nutrition:

- 273 Calories
- 14.2g Fat
- 0.7g Fiber

Seared Scallops Topped with Wasabi Mayo

Preparation Time: 10 minutes

Cooking Time: 10 minutes

Servings: 2

Ingredients:

- 1 tsp. wasabi paste
- 1 tsp. water
- 1 tbsp. butter
- 2 tbsp. mayonnaise
- 2 slices ginger (pickled, chopped)
- 8 large sea scallops
- black pepper
- chives (chopped)
- salt

Directions:

1. Combine the wasabi paste and mayonnaise and mix well to incorporate. Use a paper towel to pat the scallops dry and season with salt and pepper.

2. In a skillet, heat the butter over medium-high heat. When the butter starts to brown, add the scallops and sear for about 1 ½ minute on each side. Place the

scallops on two plates—4 scallops each—and add a dollop of wasabi mayo.

3. Finalize by topping with pickled ginger and fresh chives. Serve immediately.

Nutrition:

- 281 Calories
- 17.1g Fats
- 23.38g Protein

Lobster-Stuffed Avocado

Preparation Time: 15 minutes

Cooking Time: 5 minutes

Serving: 4

Ingredients:

- 1 tbsp. avocado oil mayonnaise
- 1 tbsp. lemon juice (fresh)
- 2 tbsp. butter (melted)
- 2 cups lobster meat (chopped, cooled at room temperature)
- 2 California avocados (halved, pitted)
- 1 celery stalk (chopped)
- 1 green onion (chopped)
- black pepper
- chives (fresh, chopped)
- salt

Directions:

1. In a bowl, combine the lobster meat, green onion, and celery. Add the mayonnaise, lemon juice, and butter, then toss lightly to coat evenly. Season with salt and pepper.
2. Use a spoon to scoop out some of the avocado flesh. Just leave about half an inch of flesh Spoon the lobster

mixture into the avocado halves—about half a cup for each. Garnish with chives and serve immediately.

Nutrition:

- 269 Calories
- 18.17g Fats
- 6.91g Carbohydrates
- 17.73g Protein

Mexican Shrimp Gazpacho

Preparation Time: 3 hours and 15 minutes

Cooking Time: 45 minutes

Serving: 4

Ingredients:

For the soup:

- ½ tsp. cumin
- 1 tbsp. balsamic vinegar
- ½ cup olive oil
- 5 ½ cups tomatoes (on the vine)
- 1 garlic clove
- 1 jalapeño
- 1 lime (juiced)
- 1 medium-sized cucumber
- 1 medium-sized red onion
- ½ red bell pepper
- sea salt

For the shrimp:

- ½ tsp. garlic powder
- ½ tsp. paprika
- ½ tsp. sea salt
- ½ tbsp. olive oil

- ½ lb. shrimp (peeled, deveined)
- For the toppings:
- 2 tbsp. cucumber (diced)
- 2 tbsp. red onion (minced)
- 2 tbsp. tomato (diced)
- 1 jalapeño (sliced thinly)
- 1 medium-sized avocado (sliced)

Directions:

1. Roughly chop the soup vegetables then place in a blender. Add the cumin, balsamic vinegar, and lime juice, then blend until you achieve a smooth consistency.
2. Keep the blender running on low, remove the lid, and pour the olive oil slowly until the consistency becomes creamy. Season with sea salt, transfer the soup to a different container, and chill for a minimum of 3 hours.
3. Prepare the shrimp right before serving the gazpacho. In a small bowl, combine all of the shrimp ingredients and toss lightly to coat evenly. Heat a skillet over medium-high heat, add the shrimps, and cook for about 3 to 4 minutes each side.
4. Take the soup out of the refrigerator, spoon into bowls, and top with the shrimp.

5. Finish it off by adding the cucumber, red onion, tomato, jalapeño, and avocado, then serve.

Nutrition:

- 12.2g Protein
- 37.2g Fat
- 445 Calories

Manhattan Clam Chowder

Preparation Time: 30 minutes

Cooking Time: 15 minutes

Serving: 8

Ingredients:

- ½ tsp. thyme (dried)
- 2 tbsp. tomato paste
- 6 tbsp. butter
- ¼ cup parsley (fresh, chopped)
- ½ cup bell pepper (diced)
- ½ cup carrot (chopped)
- ½ cup dry white wine
- ½ cup onion (diced)
- 1 cup clam juice
- 1 ¼ cup celery root (peeled, diced)
- 1 ¾ cup plum tomatoes (whole with juice)
- 2 ½ cup whole baby clams (canned with liquid)
- 4 cups chicken broth (unsalted)
- 1/3 lb. bacon (diced)
- 2 bay leaves
- 2 large garlic cloves (roughly chopped)
- black pepper
- salt

Directions:

1. Heat a soup pot over medium heat. Once hot, add a small amount of oil along with the diced bacon.

2. Cook the bacon until crispy, stirring occasionally for about 5 minutes. Turn down the heat to medium-low then add bell pepper, carrot, onion, celery root, and garlic. Continue stirring to coat the veggies with bacon grease evenly.

3. Add the wine and cover the pot. Allow the veggies to sweat for 2 to 3 minutes. Open the lid, stir, then add in the bay leaves, tomato paste, and thyme. Crush the tomatoes and add them to the pot with the liquid. Also, add the clam juice and chicken broth.

4. Turn up the heat to medium-high and bring the chowder to a boil. Once it starts boiling, return the heat to medium-low and allow the chowder to simmer for about 15 minutes. Add the clams and continue simmering. Also, add the butter and stir until melted.

5. Add salt and a lot of pepper to bring out the soup's savory flavor. Finally, stir the parsley in, then serve hot.

Nutrition:

- 15g Protein
- 36.1g Fat
- 429 Calories

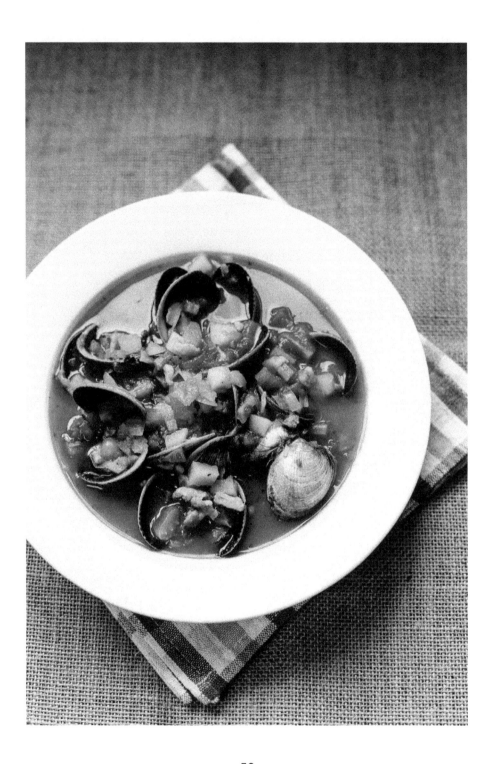

Fried Soft-Shell Crab

Preparation Time: 16 minutes

Cooking Time: 5 minutes

Serving: 2

Ingredients:

- 4 tbsp. barbecue sauce
- ½ cup lard
- ½ cup parmesan cheese (powdered)
- 2 eggs (beaten)
- 8 soft shell crabs

Directions:

1. Heat a skillet with lard over medium-high heat. Use a paper towel to pat the crabs dry. Prepare the parmesan and eggs by placing them in separate shallow dishes.
2. Dip one crab into the egg, tap off any excess, and dip into the parmesan cheese. Make sure the crab is coated well and evenly. Drop batches of crabs into the oil and cook for about 2 minutes on each side.
3. Serve the crabs hot with barbecue sauce for dipping.

Nutrition:

- 20.5g Protein
- 21.2g Fat
- 299 Calories

Convenient Tilapia Casserole

Preparation Time: 15 minutes

Cooking Time: 14 minutes

Serving: 4

Ingredients:

- 2 (14-oz.) cans sugar-free diced tomatoes with basil and garlic with juice
- 1/3 C. fresh parsley, chopped and divided
- ¼ tsp. dried oregano
- ½ tsp. red pepper flakes, crushed
- 4 (6-oz.) tilapia fillets
- 2 tbsp. fresh lemon juice
- 2/3 C. feta cheese, crumbled

Directions:

1. Preheat the oven to 400° F. In a shallow baking dish, mix tomatoes, ¼ C. of the parsley, oregano and red pepper flakes.
2. Arrange the tilapia fillets over the tomato mixture in a single layer and drizzle with the lemon juice.
3. Place some tomato mixture over the tilapia fillets and sprinkle with the feta cheese evenly. Bake for about 12-14 minutes. Serve hot with the garnishing of remaining parsley.

Nutrition:

- 246 Calories
- 9.4g Carbohydrates
- 37.2g Protein

Quick Dinner Tilapia

Preparation Time: 15 minutes

Cooking Time: 6 minutes

Servings: 5

Ingredients:

- 2 tbsp. coconut oil
- 5 (5-oz.) tilapia fillets
- 2 tbsp. unsweetened coconut, shredded
- 3 garlic cloves, minced
- 1 tbsp. fresh ginger, minced
- 2 tbsp. low-sodium soy sauce
- 8 scallions, chopped

Directions:

1. Heat up coconut oil over medium heat and cook the tilapia fillets for about 2 minutes. Flip the side and stir in the coconut, garlic and ginger.
2. Cook for about 1 minute. Add the soy sauce and cook for about 1 minute. Add the scallions and cook for about 1-2 more minutes. Remove from heat and serve hot.

Nutrition:

- 189 Calories
- 4.4g Carbohydrates
- 27.7g Protein

Hit Salmon Dinner

Preparation Time: 15 minutes

Cooking Time: 20 minutes

Servings: 2

Ingredients:

- 1 C. walnuts
- 1 tbsp. fresh dill, chopped
- 2 tbsp. fresh lemon rind, grated
- ½ tsp. garlic salt
- 1 tbsp. butter, melted
- 3-4 tbsp. Dijon mustard
- 4 (3-oz.) salmon fillets
- 4 tsp. fresh lemon juice

Directions:

1. Preheat the oven to 350° F. Line a large baking sheet with parchment paper. In a food processor, place the walnuts and pulse until chopped roughly. Add the dill, lemon rind, garlic salt, black pepper, and butter and pulse until a crumbly mixture form.

2. Place the salmon fillets onto prepared baking sheet in a single layer, skin-side down. Rub the top of each salmon fillet with Dijon mustard.

3. Place the walnut mixture over each fillet and gently, press into the surface of salmon. Bake for about 15-20 minutes. Remove the salmon fillets from oven and transfer onto the serving plates. Drizzle with the lemon juice and serve.

Nutrition:

- 691 Calories
- 10.3g Carbohydrates
- 49.8g Protein

Luscious Salmon

Preparation Time: 10 minutes

Cooking Time: 20 minutes

Servings: 2

Ingredients:

- ¼ C. cream cheese, softened
- 2 tbsp. fresh chives, chopped
- 1 tsp. garlic powder
- ¼ tsp. cayenne pepper
- 2 (4-oz.) salmon fillets

Directions:

1. Preheat the oven to 350° F. Lightly, grease a small baking dish. In a bowl, add the cream cheese, chives, spices, salt and black pepper and mix well. Arrange the salmon fillets into prepared baking dish and top with the cream cheese mixture evenly.
2. Bake for about 15-20 minutes. Remove the salmon fillets from oven and serve hot.

Nutrition:

- 257 Calories
- 2.1g Carbohydrates
- 24.6g Protein

Insanely Simple Salmon

Preparation Time: 10 minutes

Cooking Time: 14 minutes

Servings: 4

Ingredients:

- 2 garlic cloves, minced
- 1 tbsp. fresh lemon zest, grated
- 2 tbsp. butter, melted
- 2 tbsp. fresh lemon juice
- 4 (6-oz.) skinless, boneless salmon fillets
- black pepper, to taste
- Salt
- 4 tbsp. feta cheese, crumbled

Directions:

1. Preheat the grill to medium-high heat. Grease the grill grate. Incorporate all ingredients except salmon fillets and feta and mix well.
2. Add the salmon fillets and coat with garlic mixture generously.
3. Grill the salmon fillets for about 6-7 minutes per side. Serve immediately with the topping of feta.

Nutrition:

- 306 Calories
- 1.4g Carbohydrates
- 34.6g Protein

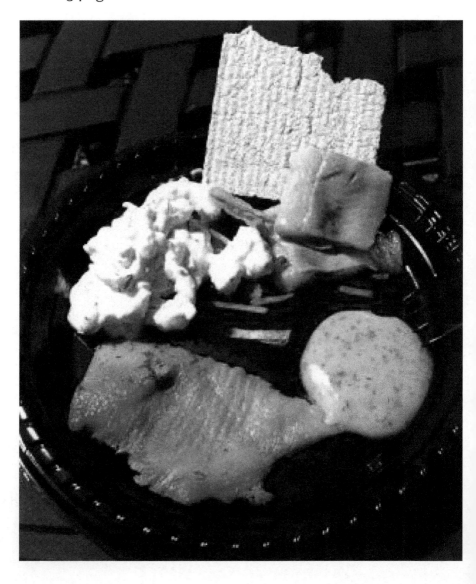

Entertaining Salmon

Preparation Time: 20 minutes

Cooking Time: 16 minutes

Servings: 4

Ingredients:

For Salmon:

- 4 (6-oz.) skinless salmon fillets
- 2 tbsp. fresh lemon juice
- 2 tbsp. olive oil, divided
- 1 tbsp. unsalted butter

For Filling:

- 4 oz. cream cheese, softened
- ¼ C. Parmesan cheese, grated finely
- 4 oz. frozen spinach thawed and squeezed
- 2 tsp. garlic, minced

Directions:

1. Season each salmon fillet then, drizzle with lemon juice and 1 tbsp. of oil. Arrange the salmon fillets onto a smooth surface.
2. With a sharp knife, cut a pocket into each salmon fillet about ¾ of the way through.

3. For filling: in a bowl, add the cream cheese, Parmesan cheese, spinach, garlic, salt and black pepper and mix well.

4. Place about 1-2 tbsp. of spinach mixture into each salmon pocket and spread evenly.

5. In a skillet, heat the remaining oil and butter over medium-high heat and cook the salmon fillets for about 6-8 minutes per side.

6. Remove the salmon fillets from heat and transfer onto the serving plates. Serve.

Nutrition:

- 438 Calories
- 2.4g Carbohydrates
- 38.1g Protein

Flavors Infused Salmon

Preparation Time: 15 minutes

Cooking Time: 15 minutes

Servings: 2

Ingredients:

- 2 (6-oz.) salmon fillets
- 2 streaky bacon slices
- 4 tbsp. pesto

Directions:

1. Preheat the oven to 350° F. Line a medium baking sheet with parchment paper. Wrap each salmon fillet with 1 bacon slice and then, secure with a wooden skewer.
2. Place 2 tbsp. of pesto in the center of each salmon fillet. Arrange the salmon fillets onto prepared baking sheet. Bake for about 15 minutes.
3. Remove the salmon fillets from oven and serve hot.

Nutrition:

- 517 Calories
- 2.4g Carbohydrates
- 46.7g Protein:

Tuna Fish Salad

Preparation Time: 5 minutes

Cooking Time: 10 minutes Servings: 1

Ingredient:

- 10 kalamata olives, pitted
- 1 small zucchini sliced lengthwise
- ½ diced avocado
- 2 cups of mixed greens
- 1 large diced tomato
- 1 sliced green onion
- 1 can chunk light tuna in water
- ¼ cup fresh parsley, chopped
- ½ cup fresh mint, chopped
- 1 tbsp. extra virgin olive oil
- 1 tbsp. balsamic vinegar
- ¼ tsp. fine sea salt
- ¾ tsp. black pepper, cracked

Directions:

1. Grill the zucchini slices on each side for a few minutes or as desired. Once cooked, cut it into bite-size pieces. Grab a large bowl and just put all the ingredients together in the container, mixing them together.

2. Serve while still fresh. This salad would taste best if eaten immediately so try not to have any leftovers.

Nutrition:

- 563 calories
- 30.9g total fat
- 37.5g carbohydrates

Mozzarella Tuna Melt

Preparation Time: 10 minutes

Cooking Time: 10 minutes Serving: 2

Ingredients:

- 1 tablespoon olive oil
- 1/2 cup diced yellow onion
- 8 ounces canned tuna
- 1/4 cup mayonnaise
- 2 large eggs
- 2 ounces shredded mozzarella cheese
- 1 green onion

Directions:

1. Warm-up oil in a skillet over medium heat. Cook onion for 5 minutes.
2. Strain the tuna then flake it into the skillet and stir in remaining ingredients.
3. Season well and cook for 2 minutes or until the cheese melts. Top with sliced green onion to serve.

Nutrition:

- 110 calories
- 10g fat
- 26g protein

Crabmeat Egg Scramble with White Sauce

Preparation Time: 10 minutes

Cooking Time: 15 minutes

Serving: 2

Ingredients:

- 1 tbsp. olive oil
- 4 eggs
- 4 oz. crabmeat

Sauce:

- ¾ cup crème fraiche
- ½ cup chives, chopped
- ½ tsp. garlic powder

Directions:

1. Scourge eggs with a fork in a bowl, and season with salt and black pepper.
2. Set a sauté pan over medium heat and warm olive oil. Add in the eggs and scramble them.
3. Stir in crabmeat and cook until cooked thoroughly. In a mixing dish, combine crème fraiche and garlic powder. Season with salt and sprinkle with chives. Serve the eggs with the white sauce.

Nutrition:

- 105 calories
- 9g fat
- 31g protein

Tuna Pickle Boats

Preparation Time: 40 minutes

Cooking Time: 0 minute

Serving: 4

Ingredients

- 1 (5-oz) can tuna, drained
- 2 large dill pickles
- ¼ tsp. lemon juice
- 2 tsp. mayonnaise
- ¼ tbsp. onion flakes
- 1 tsp. dill. chopped

Directions:

1. Cut the pickles in half lengthwise. Spoon out the seeds to create boats; set aside.
2. Combine the mayonnaise, tuna, onion flakes, and lemon juice in a bowl. Fill each boat with tuna mixture. Sprinkle with dill and place in the fridge for 30 minutes before serving.

Nutrition:

- 311 calories
- 12g fat
- 4g protein

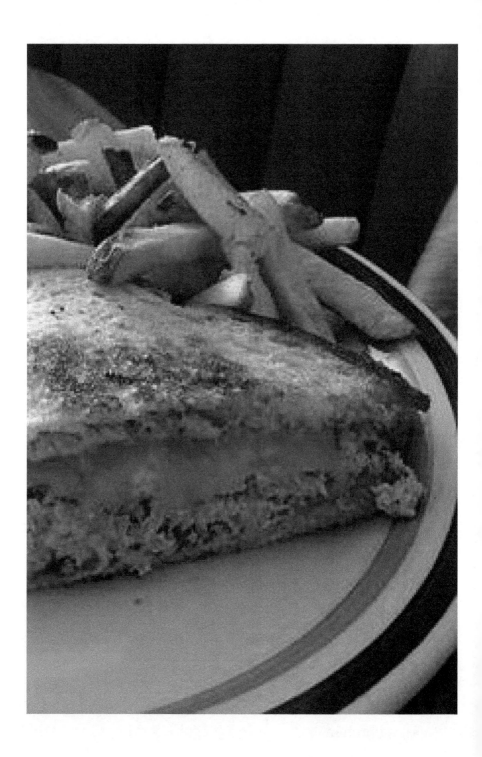

Salmon Salad with Lettuce & Avocado

Preparation Time: 5 minutes

Cooking Time: 0 minute

Serving: 3

Ingredients:

- 2 slices smoked salmon
- 1 tsp. onion flakes
- 3 tbsp. mayonnaise
- 1 cup romaine lettuce
- 1 tbsp. lime juice
- 1 tbsp. extra virgin olive oil
- ½ avocado, sliced

Directions:

1. Combine the salmon, mayonnaise, lime juice, olive oil, and salt in a small bowl; mix to combine well.
2. In a salad platter, arrange the shredded lettuce and onion flakes. Spread the salmon mixture over; top with avocado slices and serve.

Nutrition:

- 112 calories
- 6g fat
- 28g protein

Mackerel Lettuce Cups

Preparation Time: 10 minutes

Cooking Time: 20 minutes

Serving: 4

Ingredients:

- 2 mackerel fillets
- 1 tbsp. olive oil
- 2 eggs
- 1 ½ cups water
- 1 tomato, seeded
- 2 tbsp. mayonnaise
- ½ head green lettuce

Directions:

1. Preheat a grill pan over medium heat. Dash mackerel fillets with olive oil, and sprinkle with salt and black pepper. Add the fish to the preheated grill pan and cook on both sides for 6-8 minutes.

2. Bring the eggs to boil in salted water in a pot over medium heat for 10 minutes. Then, run the eggs in cold water, peel, and chop into small pieces. Transfer to a salad bowl.

3. Remove the mackerel fillets to the salad bowl. Include the tomatoes and mayonnaise; mix evenly with a spoon.

4. Layer two lettuce leaves each as cups and fill with two tablespoons of egg salad each.

Nutrition:

- 107 calories
- 14g fat
- 27g protein

Chicken-of-Sea Salad

Preparation Time: 15 minutes

Cooking Time: 5 minutes

Servings: 6

Ingredients:

- 2 (6-oz.) cans olive oil-packed tuna
- 2 (6-oz.) cans water packed tuna
- ¾ C. mayonnaise
- 2 celery stalks
- ¼ of onion
- 1 tbsp. fresh lime juice
- 2 tbsp. mustard
- 6 C. fresh baby arugula

Directions:

1. In a large bowl, add all the ingredients except arugula and gently stir to combine. Divide arugula onto serving plates and top with tuna mixture. Serve immediately.

Nutrition:

- 325 Calories
- 27.4g Protein
- 1.1g Fiber

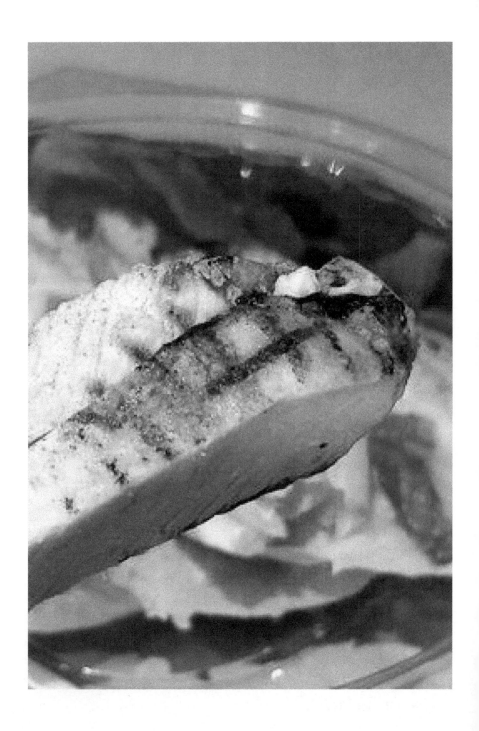

Smoked Salmon Salad

Preparation Time: 17 minutes

Cooking Time: 10 minutes

Servings: 4

Ingredients:

- 8 oz. smoked salmon, sliced into thin pieces
- 2 oz. pecans, crushed
- 3 medium tomatoes, chopped
- ½ cup lettuce, chopped
- 1 cucumber, diced
- 1/3 cup cream cheese
- 1/3 cup coconut milk
- ½ tsp. oregano
- 1 tbsp. lemon juice, chopped
- ½ tsp. basil
- 1 tsp. salt

Directions:

1. In medium bowl, combine salmon with pecans and stir. Add tomatoes, lettuce and cucumber, stir well.
2. In another bowl, mix together cream cheese, coconut milk, oregano, lemon juice, basil and salt. Stir mixture until get homogenous mass. Serve salmon salad with cream cheese sauce.

Nutrition:

- 211 Calories
- 15.9g Fat
- 9.95g Protein

Tuna Salad

Preparation Time: 18 minutes

Cooking Time: 10 minutes

Servings: 4

Ingredients:

- 1 can tuna
- 4 eggs, boiled, peeled and chopped
- 1 oz. olives, pitted and sliced
- 1/3 cup cheese cream
- ½ cup almond milk
- ½ tsp. ground black pepper
- ½ tsp. kosher salt
- 1 tbsp. garlic, minced

Directions:

1. In medium bowl, mash tuna with fork. Add chopped eggs and stir. Add sliced olives and stir.
2. In another bowl, whisk together cheese cream and almond milk. Add black pepper, salt and garlic, stir carefully. Add cheese mixture to tuna mixture and mix up. Serve.

Nutrition:

- 182 Calories

- 11.9g Fat
- 12.88g Protein

Smoked Salmon and Goat Cheese Bites

Preparation Time: 10 minutes

Cooking Time: 15 minutes

Servings: 16

Ingredients:

- 8 ounces goat cheese, softened
- 1 tablespoon fresh oregano
- 1 tablespoon fresh rosemary
- 1 tablespoon fresh basil
- 2 cloves garlic
- Salt and pepper to taste
- 6 ounces radicchio
- 4 ounces smoked salmon

Directions:

1. Finely mince the oregano, rosemary, and fresh basil. Finely grate the garlic. Add the goat cheese, herbs, garlic, salt, and pepper to a mixing bowl. Combine well then set aside.

2. Cut the stem off the bottom of the radicchio. Carefully peel apart the leaves until you have 16 leaves for serving. You can save any leftover radicchio for other salads or recipes. Wash the leaves then dry them.

3. On each radicchio leave lay a piece of smoked salmon then a ½ ounce of the herbed goat cheese. Sprinkle some black pepper across the top then serve.

Nutrition:

- 46.19 Calories
- 3.33g Fats
- 3.43g Protein.

Loaded Cauliflower Mashed "Potatoes"

Preparation Time: 4 minutes

Cooking Time: 10 minutes

Servings: 4

Ingredients:

- 1 head fresh cauliflower, cut into cubes
- 2 garlic cloves, minced
- 6 tablespoons butter
- 2 tablespoons sour cream
- Pink Himalayan salt
- Freshly ground black pepper
- 1 cup shredded cheese (I use Colby Jack)
- 6 bacon slices, cooked and crumbled

Directions:

1. Boil a large pot of water over high heat. Add the cauliflower. Reduce the heat to medium-low and simmer for 8 to 10 minutes, until fork-tender. (You can also steam the cauliflower if you have a steamer basket.)

2. Drain the cauliflower in a colander, and turn it out onto a paper towel lined plate to soak up the water. Blot to remove any remaining water from the cauliflower pieces. This step is important; you want to

get out as much water as possible so the mash won't be runny.

3. Add the cauliflower to the food processor (or blender) with the garlic, butter, and sour cream, and season with pink Himalayan salt and pepper. Mix for about 1 minute, stopping to scrape down the sides of the bowl every 30 seconds.

4. Divide the cauliflower mix evenly among four small serving dishes, and top each with the cheese and bacon crumbles. (The cheese should melt from the hot cauliflower. But if you want to reheat it, you can put the cauliflower in oven-safe serving dishes and pop them under the broiler for 1 minute to heat up the cauliflower and melt the cheese.) Serve warm.

Nutrition:

- 757 Calories
- 38g Total Fat
- 6g Fiber
- 29g Protein

Keto Bread

Preparation Time: 5 minutes

Cooking Time: 25 minutes

Servings: 6

Ingredients:

- 5 tablespoons butter, at room temperature, divided
- 6 large eggs, lightly beaten
- 1½ cups almond flour
- 3 teaspoons baking powder
- 1 scoop MCT oil powder
- Pinch pink Himalayan salt

Directions:

1. Preheat the oven to 390°F. Coat a 9-by-5-inch loaf pan with 1 tablespoon of butter. In a large bowl, use a hand mixer to mix the eggs, almond flour, remaining 4 tablespoons of butter, baking powder, MCT oil powder (if using), and pink Himalayan salt until thoroughly blended. Pour into the prepared pan.
2. Bake for 25 minutes, or until a toothpick inserted in the center comes out clean. Slice and serve.

Nutrition:

- 165 Calories
- 15g Total Fat
- 2g Fiber
- 6g Protein

Keto Tortilla Chips

Preparation Time: 5 minutes

Cooking Time: 5 minutes

Servings: 36 pieces

Ingredients:

Tortilla Chips:

- 6 flax seed tortillas
- 3 tbsp. Oil for deep frying, (absorbed oil)
- Salt and pepper to taste

Toppings:

- Diced jalapeno
- Fresh salsa
- Shredded cheese
- Full-fat sour cream

Directions:

1. Make the flaxseed tortilla's using this recipe. I get 6 total tortillas when using a tortilla press.
2. Cut the tortillas into chip-sized slices. I got 6 out of each tortilla.
3. Heat the deep fryer. Once ready, lay out the pieces of tortilla in the basket. You can fry 4-6 pieces at a time.

Fry for about 1-2 minutes, then flip. Continue to fry for another 1-2 minutes on the other side.

4. Remove from the fryer and place on paper towels to cool. Season with salt and pepper to taste. Serve with toppings of choice!

Nutrition:

- 40.34 Calories
- 3.03g Fats
- 0.37g Net Carbs
- 0.83g Protein.

Flavored Keto Cheese Chips

Preparation Time: 10 minutes

Cooking Time: 5 minutes

Servings: 15

Ingredients:

- 1 ½ cups shredded cheddar cheese
- 3 tablespoons ground flaxseed meal
- Seasonings of Your Choice

Directions:

1. Preheat your oven to 425°F. Start by forming 2 Tbsp. Cheddar Cheese into small mounds on your non-stick pan. You want to spread them out a little bit as they will melt and expand as they're cooking.

2. In a small ramekin, measure out 3 Tbsp. Flaxseed Meal. Use this to distribute the flax evenly among all the chips you're making. Add the seasonings of your choice to the chips! In this batch we're making 3 different flavors.

3. The first flavor is paprika and cumin. I have large spice containers for these 2, as I use them a lot. I poured them straight onto the chip and probably used more than I should have. Lesson learned: sprinkle the spices on with your fingers.

4. The second flavor is southwest chipotle and cheddar. I am using Tone's Southwest Chipotle Seasoning, one that I think is a must-have in every pantry.

5. The third, and last, flavor is a blend of onion powder, garlic powder, chili, celery seed and a few others.

6. Once all the chips are seasoned to your liking, put them in the oven for 10 minutes. They shouldn't look crisp when you take them out, but you will see little holes forming in the chips where the oil is pooling on the top.

7. Remove the chips from the oven and let them cool for 1-2 minutes. They'll start to get hard and form into the crispy chips we want. If you want to form them into different shapes, you can do that here – but be quick!

8. Transfer the chips to a paper towel to quickly get rid of excess grease. Once finished, transfer them to a platter plate. You can put salsa in the middle and serve as an appetizer or snack.

Nutrition:

- 65.83 Calories
- 5.27g Fats
- 3.61g Protein.

Smoked Salmon and Goat Cheese Bites

Preparation Time: 10 minutes

Cooking Time: 15 minutes

Servings: 16

Ingredients:

- 8 ounces goat cheese, softened
- 1 tablespoon fresh oregano
- 1 tablespoon fresh rosemary
- 1 tablespoon fresh basil
- 2 cloves garlic
- Salt and pepper to taste
- 6 ounces radicchio
- 4 ounces smoked salmon

Directions:

4. Finely mince the oregano, rosemary, and fresh basil. Finely grate the garlic. Add the goat cheese, herbs, garlic, salt, and pepper to a mixing bowl. Combine well then set aside.

5. Cut the stem off the bottom of the radicchio. Carefully peel apart the leaves until you have 16 leaves for serving. You can save any leftover radicchio for other salads or recipes. Wash the leaves then dry them.

6. On each radicchio leave lay a piece of smoked salmon then a ½ ounce of the herbed goat cheese. Sprinkle some black pepper across the top then serve.

Nutrition:

- 46.19 Calories
- 3.33g Fats
- 3.43g Protein.

Low Carb Fried Mac & Cheese

Preparation Time: 5 minutes

Cooking Time: 10 minutes

Servings: 5

Ingredients:

- 1 medium cauliflower, riced
- 1 ½ cups shredded cheddar cheese
- 3 large eggs
- 2 teaspoons paprika
- 1 teaspoon turmeric
- ¾ teaspoon rosemary

Directions:

1. Get your head of cauliflower ready. We'll need to prep it before ricing it. Cut your cauliflower into florets, making sure you get any excess stem off. Add the cauliflower to your food processor and pulse it until it is the consistency of short grain rice. Put your cauliflower into a microwave safe bowl, and microwave for 5-7 minutes.

2. Once it's done in the microwave, we want to get all the excess moisture out. I lay my cauliflower onto a kitchen towel to wring it out. You will get cauliflower "juice" all over the towel, so this will need to go into

the laundry afterward. If you don't want to do that, you can do this with paper towels also.

3. Once you have the cauliflower in the kitchen towel, roll it up tight and apply pressure (your whole-body weight) to the cauliflower. Try to push as much extra moisture out of the cauliflower as you can.

4. Once you're finished, extract the "mushed" cauliflower from the kitchen towel and put it into a bowl. Make sure that its room temperature by this point.

5. Add your eggs ONE AT A TIME to the cauliflower. You don't want a mixture that too watery! Keep in mind that I only did 1/3 of the entire recipe. Add your cheese.

6. Finally, your spices to the cauliflower – turmeric, rosemary, and paprika. Mix everything well, using your hands if you want.

7. In a pan, heat your olive oil and coconut oil on high until it gets very hot. Form your cauliflower mixture into a ball, and then flatten it out in the palm of your hand. Add your cauliflower "patties" into the hot oil and reduce the heat to medium high.

8. Allow them to get crisp on one side before flipping them. Continue cooking them until they're crisp on both sides. All done! Serve on a bed of spinach, or just eat as a snack. They're absolutely delicious!

Nutrition:

- 39.67 Calories
- 2.71g Fats
- 2.59g Protein.

Feta and Bacon Bites

Preparation Time: 10 minutes

Cooking Time: 15 minutes

Servings: 24

Ingredients:

- ¾ cup almond flour
- 2 cups mozzarella cheese, shredded
- 8 slices cooked bacon
- ¼ cup feta cheese, crumbled
- ¼ cup green onions, chopped
- 3 tablespoons sriracha mayo, like Sarayo
- Salt and pepper to taste

Directions:

1. Preheat your oven to 350°F. In a nonstick pan over medium heat, combine your almond flour and mozzarella. Stir constantly. Your flour/cheese mix will form a dough like consistency after about 5 minutes.

2. Place your dough between two pieces of parchment paper. Roll flat with a rolling pin. Use a cookie cutter or glass to cut out 24 circles.

3. If you run out of dough then form the remaining bits into a ball. Heat it up on stove, then roll it out again.

4. Place the circles of dough into your muffin tin (or on a cookie sheet.) Top with the bacon, feta, and onions. Bake at 350°F for about 15 minutes, until the edges are browned. Cool, peel off the liners, and top with sriracha mayo!

Nutrition:

- 71.79 Calories
- 5.74g Fats
- 3.66g Protein.

Low Carb Flax Bread

Preparation Time: 10 minutes

Cooking Time: 20 minutes

Servings: 8

Ingredients:

- 200 g ground flax seeds
- ½ cup psyllium husk powder
- 1 tablespoon baking powder
- 1 ½ cups soy protein isolate
- ¼ cup granulated Stevia
- 2 teaspoons salt
- 7 large egg whites
- 1 large whole egg
- 3 tablespoons butter
- ¾ cup water

Directions:

1. Preheat oven to 350°F. Mix psyllium husk, baking powder, protein isolate, sweetener, and salt together.
2. In a separate bowl, mix the egg, egg whites, butter, and water together. If you decide to add extracts or syrups, add these here! Slowly add wet ingredients to dry ingredients while mixing them.

3. Grease bread pan. Add all ingredients to the bread pan. Bake for 15-20 minutes until set.

Nutrition:

- 265.5 Calories
- 15.68g Fats
- 24.34g Protein.

Crispy & Delicious Kale Chips

Preparation Time: 5 minutes

Cooking Time: 15 minutes

Servings: 8

Ingredients:

- 1 large bunch kale
- 2 tablespoons olive oil
- 1 tablespoon seasoned salt

Directions:

1. Preheat your oven to 350°F. Remove your bindings on your bunch of kale. Separate the leaves from the stems of your kale. You want to try to get as little stem as possible. Rinse your kale with cold water. Add it to your vegetable spinner and remove as much water as possible.

2. Add your kale to a kitchen towel and remove excess water drops. Put your kale into a Ziploc bag and add 1 Tbsp. Olive Oil. Mix it well so that it coats every single leaf.

3. Add your kale to a baking sheet. You want to make sure that the kale is spread out a little bit. Try to press the leaves flat so you get a more even and crisped cook on each leaf.

4. Bake the kale for 12 minutes and remove from the oven. You want the edges of the kale to be a little browned, but the rest of the kale to stay a darkish green.

5. BE CAREFUL – there is a fine line between being overcooked and being perfect. When they're overcooked, they come out very bitter.

6. Add your salt to the finished kale and serve! You can add different seasonings, or just use your favorite seasoned salt.

Nutrition:

- 80.5 Calories
- 7.15g Fats
- 1.82g Protein.